Tommy's Tonsil Tales

Little Med Minds Series

Written By: Christopher Kruglik and Josephine Yalovitser
Illustrations By: Josephine Yalovitser

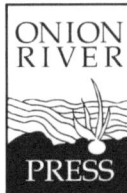

ONION
RIVER
PRESS

Burlington, Vermont

Onion River Press
89 Church Street
Burlington, VT 05401

info@onionriverpress.com
www.onionriverpress.com

ISBN: 978-1-966607-29-8
Library of Congress Control Number: 2025915943

We dedicate this book in memory of Dr. Laurence Coffin, a Vermont heart surgeon and painter whose creativity and accomplishments continue to inspire projects like this one. His legacy lives on through family and friends who carry on his mission to bridge arts and medicine, improving patient education and outcomes through creative and compassionate innovation.

With heartfelt thanks to Dr. Richard N. Hubbell, whose wise guidance and kind support helped bring this story to life.

Little Med Minds Series: Tommy's Tonsil Tales

If you're ready for a tonsil-tastic adventure, come jump into **Tommy's Tonsil Tales**—a special edition from the *Little Med Minds* series! Follow Tommy as he discovers why tonsils sometimes need to go, how doctors can help, and what happens during and after the procedure where his tonsils and adenoids are removed.

Little Med Minds is here to:

- Teach kids about their bodies and health in fun and easy ways
- Give kids superpowers like bravery and curiosity, so they can take an active role in their own care
- Answer questions that kids might have about hospitals, check-ups, and more
- Help turn scary moments, like doctor visits or procedures, into exciting learning adventures
- Build trust between children and their doctors
- Spark a love for medicine and science through memorable stories

In this story led by Tommy, kids will:

- Learn how tonsils work and why some need to be removed
- See how doctors and families team up to keep people healthy
- Explore what happens at the hospital during this procedure (Spoiler: It's not scary with Tommy around!)

For Parents & Caregivers:

This book is a tool to start conversations, ease worries, and empower your child. While Tommy's journey teaches kids important lessons about their health, always consult your healthcare provider for medical advice.

Do you love learning with Tommy?

Explore more *Little Med Minds* stories to grow your child's curiosity and confidence! Available where all books are sold.

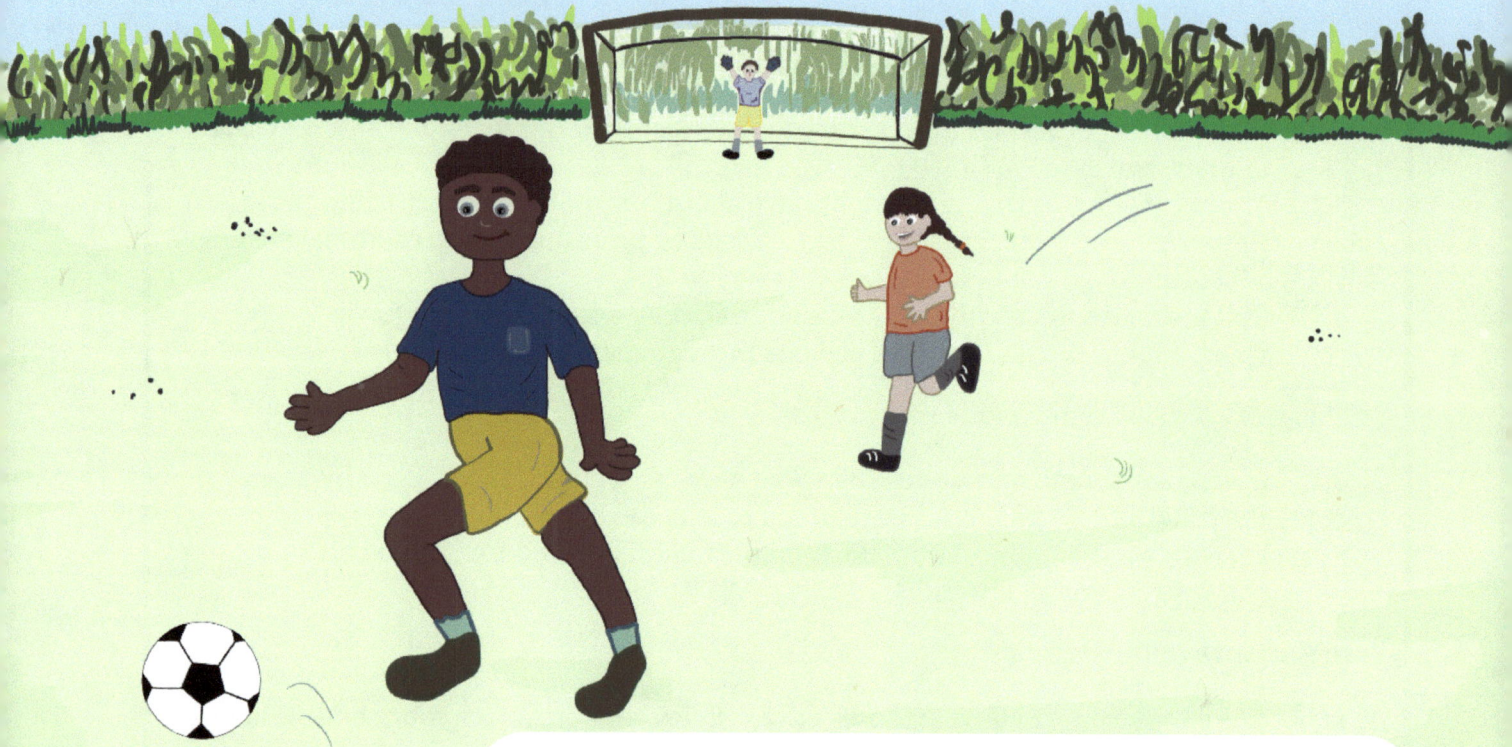

Once upon a time, in a town not so small,
lived a boy named Tommy, the most lively of all.
He laughed and he played with his friends in the sun,
but his throat often hurt, which really spoiled his fun.

Seven times one year, Tommy fell ill with strep,
it made him feel nauseous with a swollen neck.
He'd take his medicine to stay right on track,
but his strep throats just seemed to keep coming back.

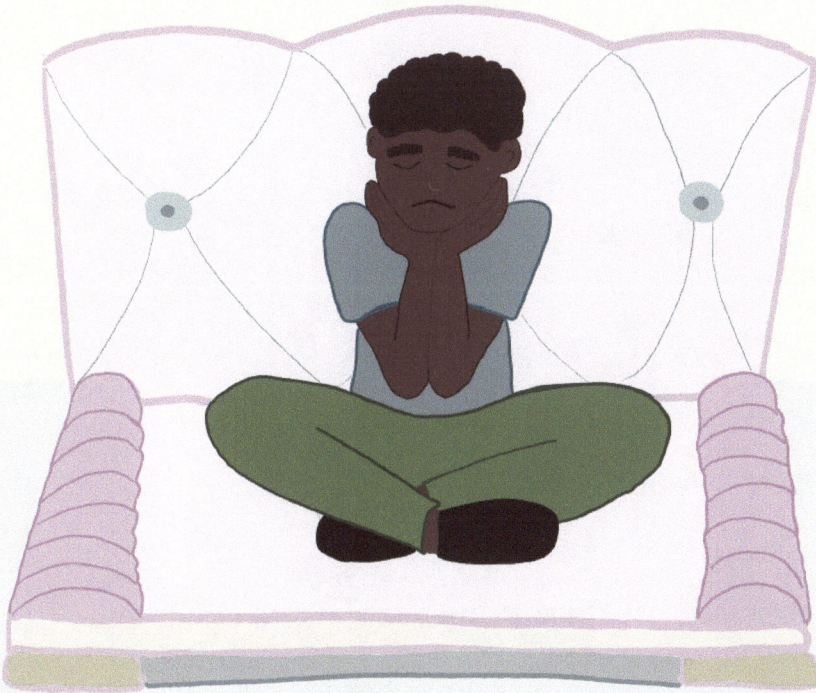

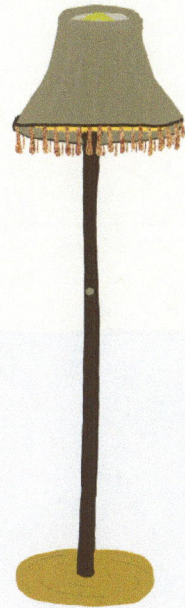

Tommy often snored as loud as a bear.

His sleep was choppy—it didn't seem fair!

He'd wake up each morning, feeling not at all peppy.

His big tonsils made breathing seem oh so schleppy.

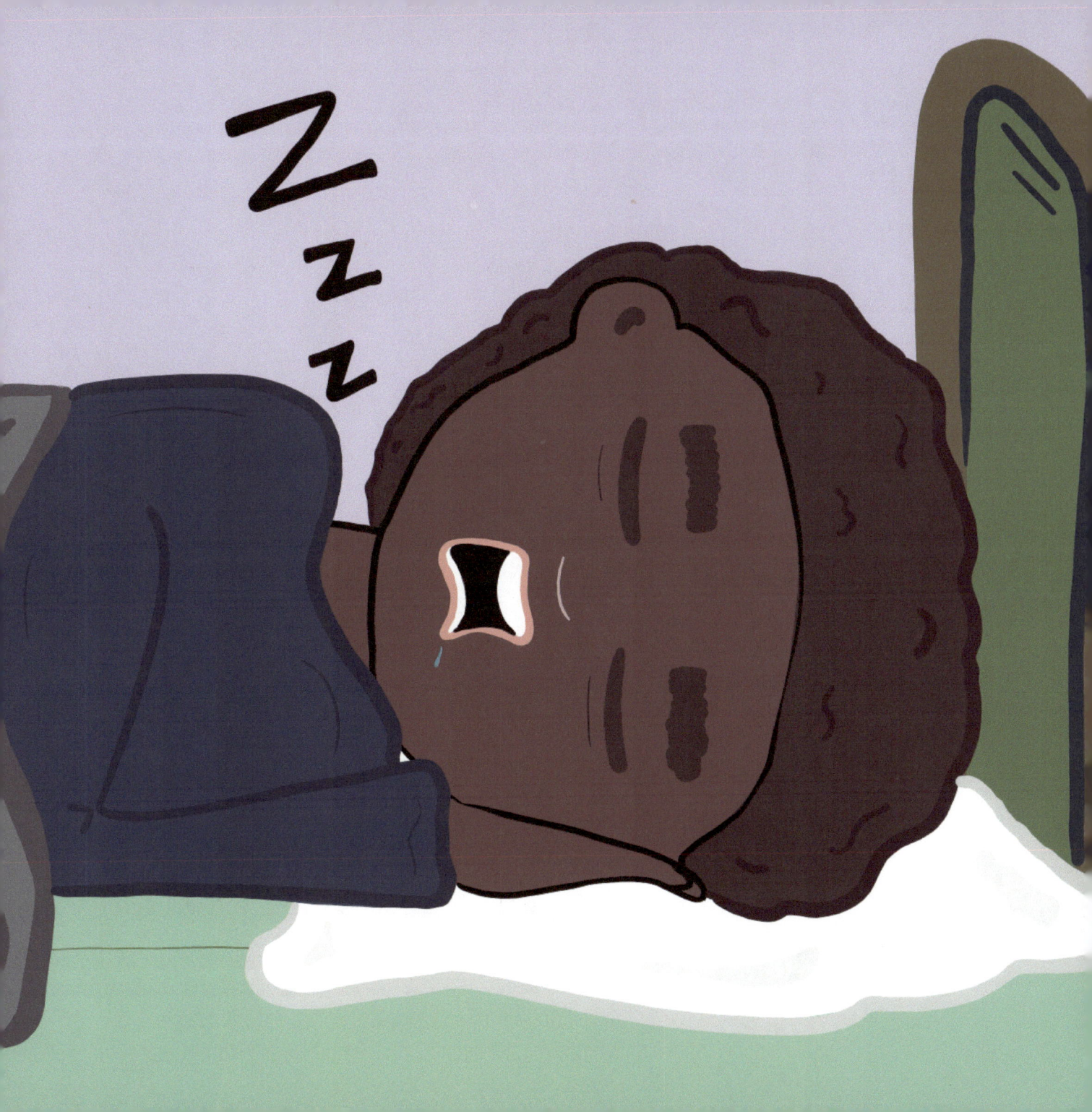

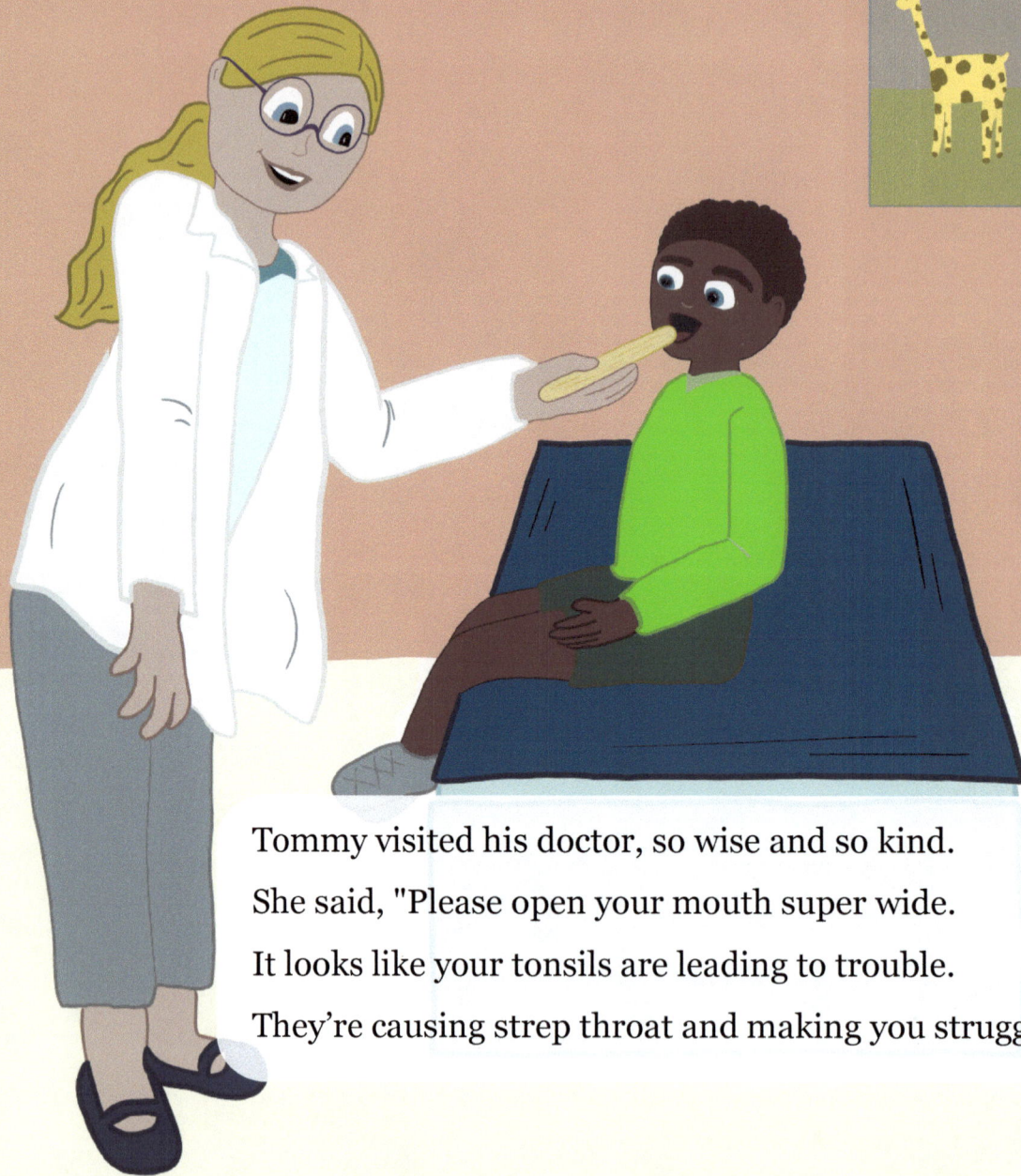

Tommy visited his doctor, so wise and so kind.

She said, "Please open your mouth super wide.

It looks like your tonsils are leading to trouble.

They're causing strep throat and making you struggle!"

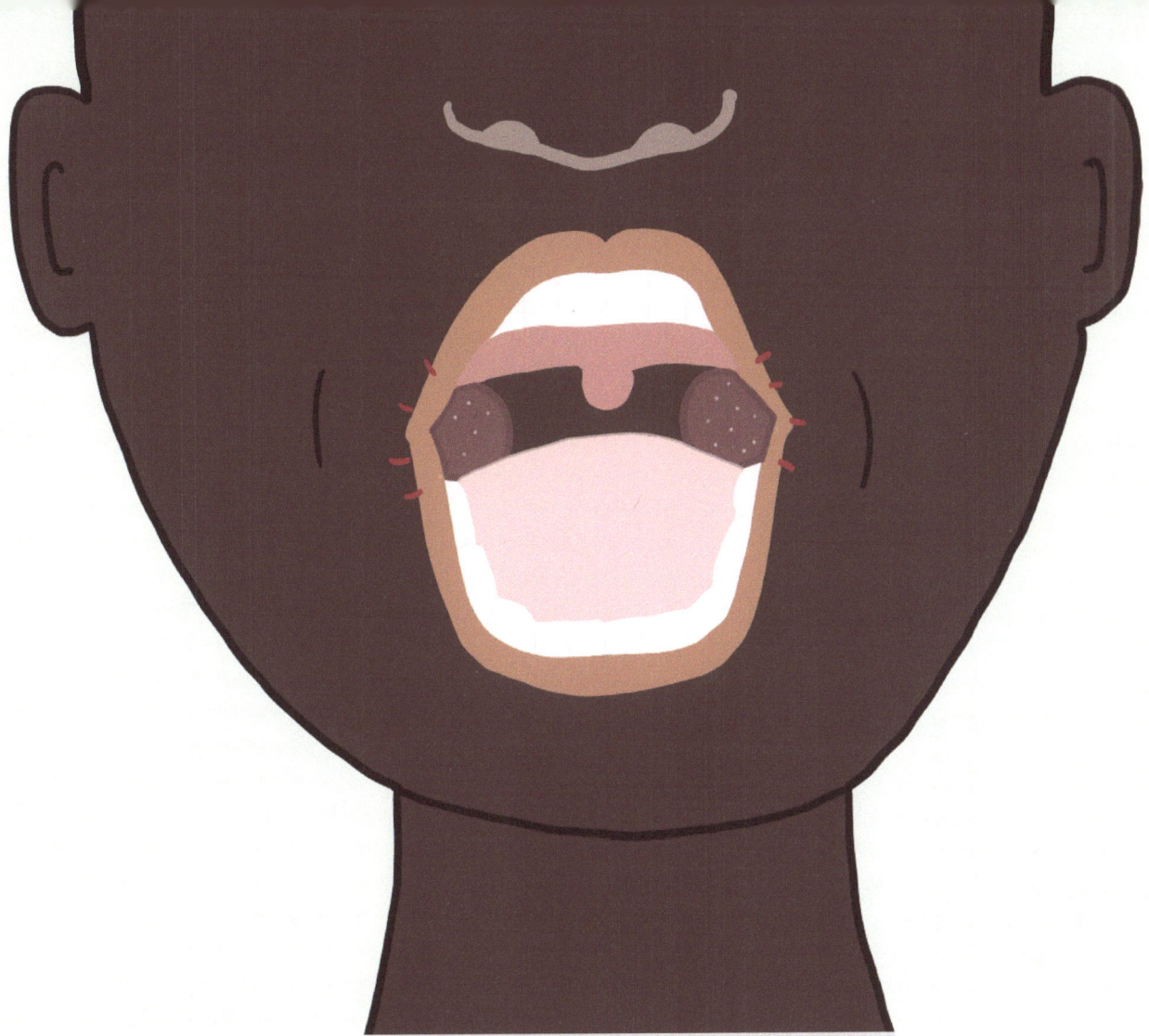

"When you fall asleep, they should let air flow free,
but yours are quite swollen and large, as I see.
They cause you to snore, and your sleep isn't sound,
and that's why you're tired, no strength to be found."

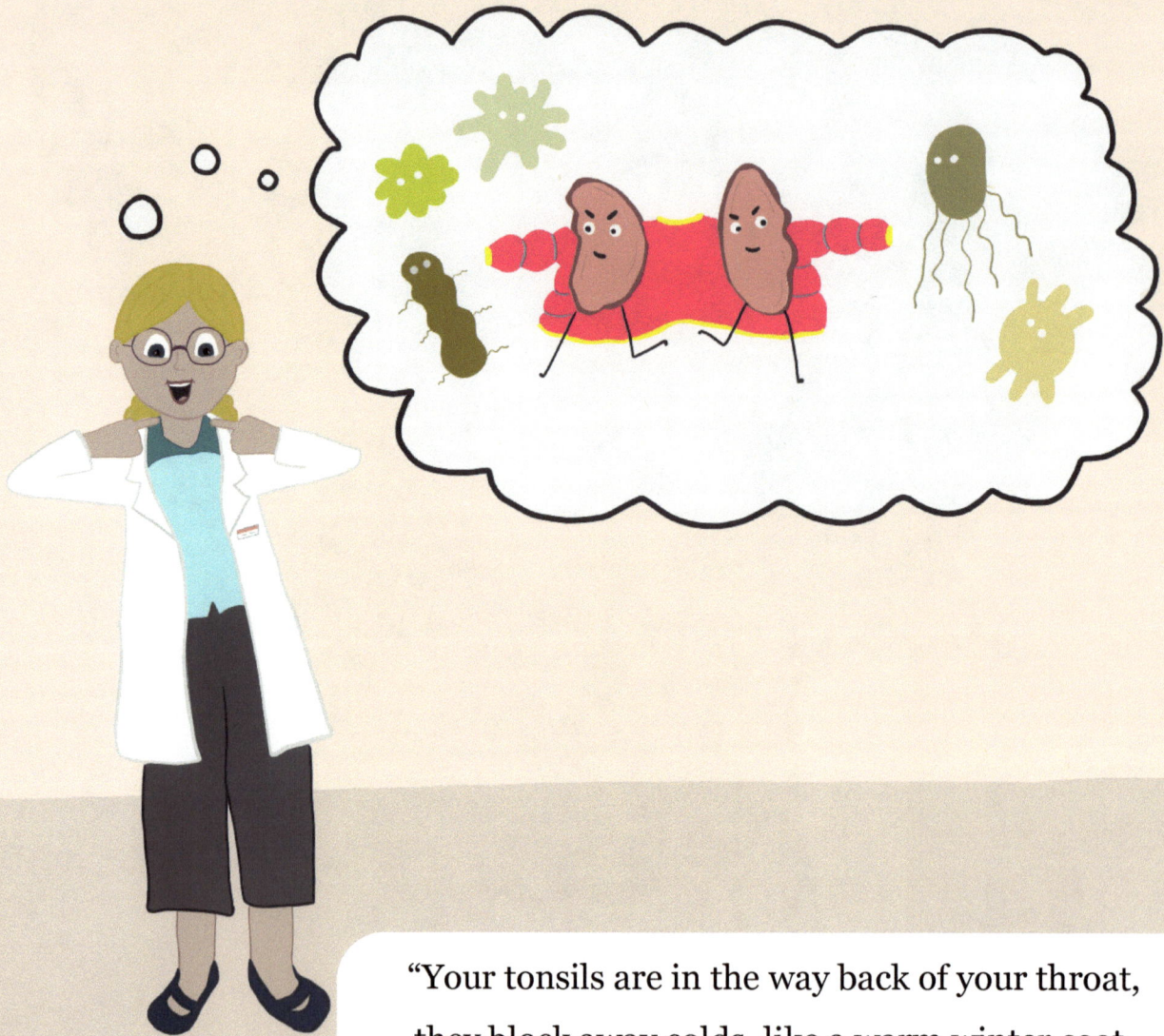

"Your tonsils are in the way back of your throat,
they block away colds, like a warm winter coat.
But yours are too big, causing trouble and pain,
we'll take them out gently and relieve all your strain.

Some kids get sore throats, over and over, it's true,
Seven times in one year, or maybe five in two.
Three times each year, after three years pass by,
is a hint that those tonsils might soon say goodbye."

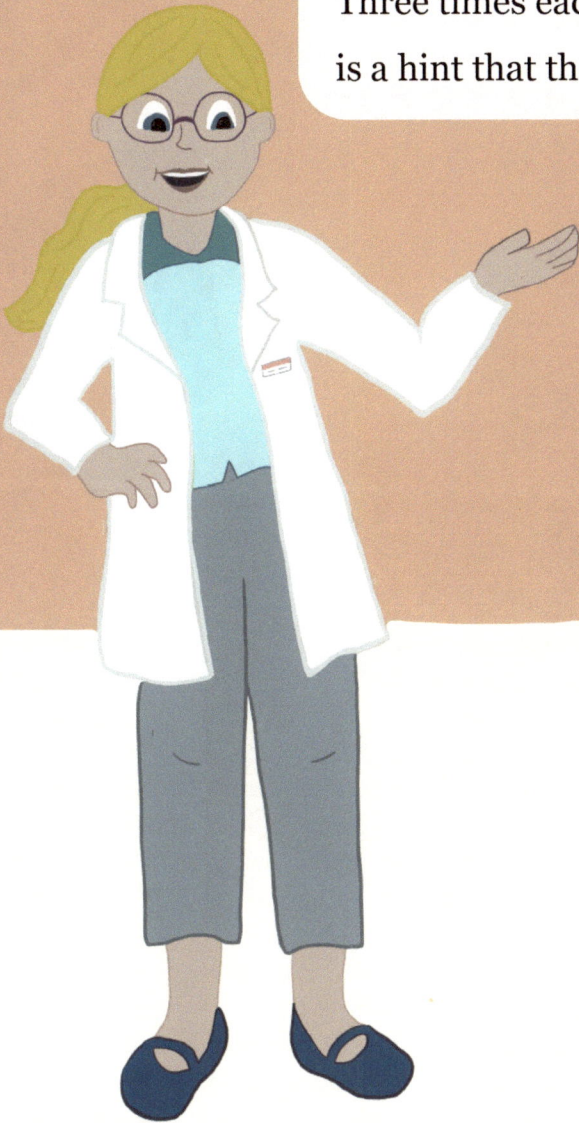

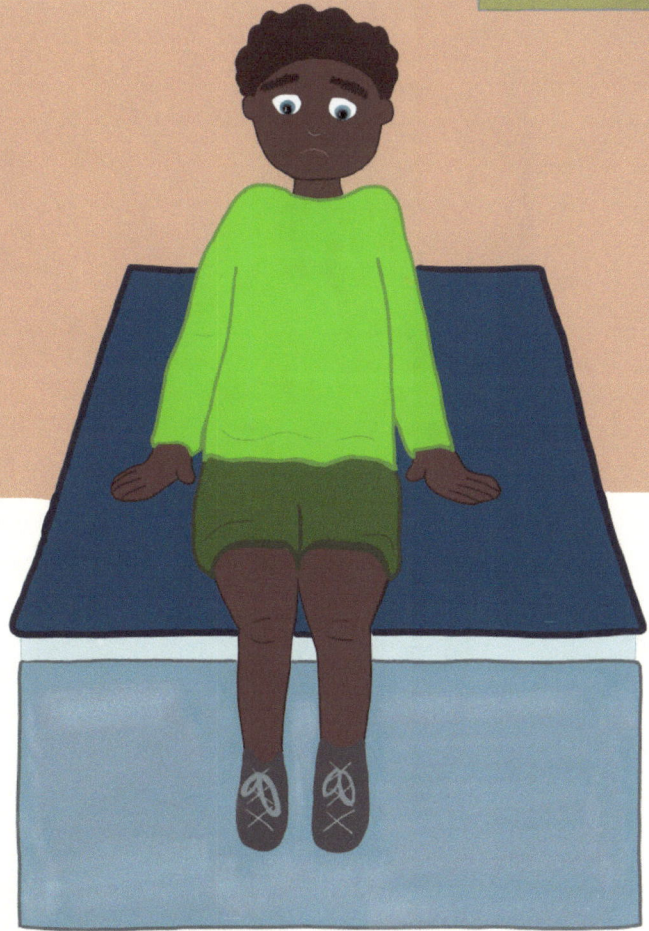

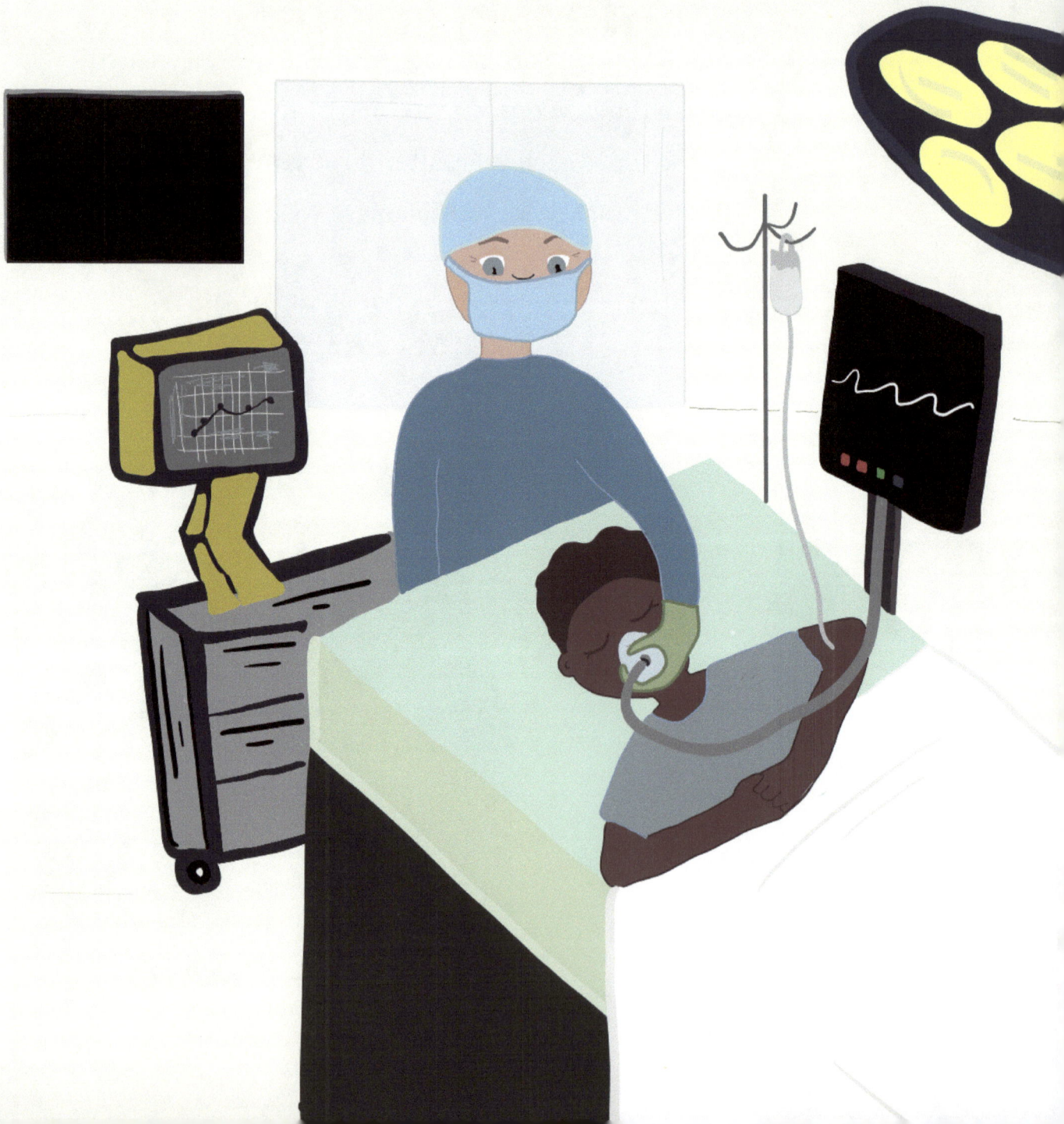

In the operating room, so bright and so neat,
Tommy lay down, snug under the sheet.
The doctors and nurses moved gently with grace,
as a voice said, "Count down, you're in a safe place...
Start from three, Let's go nice and slow."
Tommy began feeling calm from his head to his toe.
"Three, two, one—" Into deep sleep he slid,
to dreamland he drifted, as one happy kid.

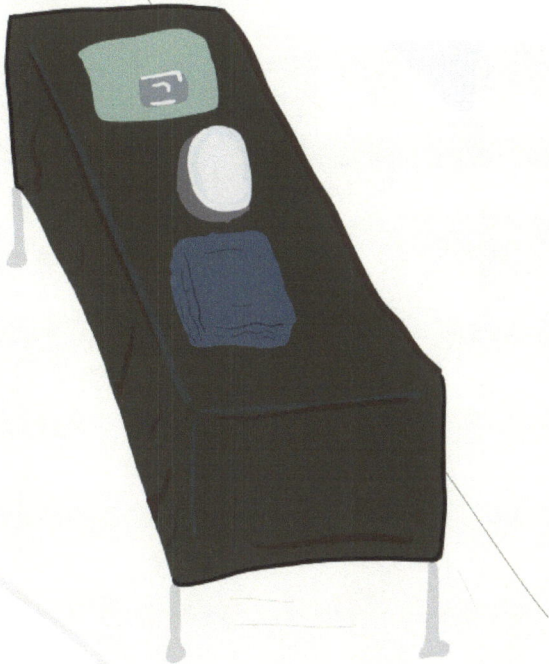

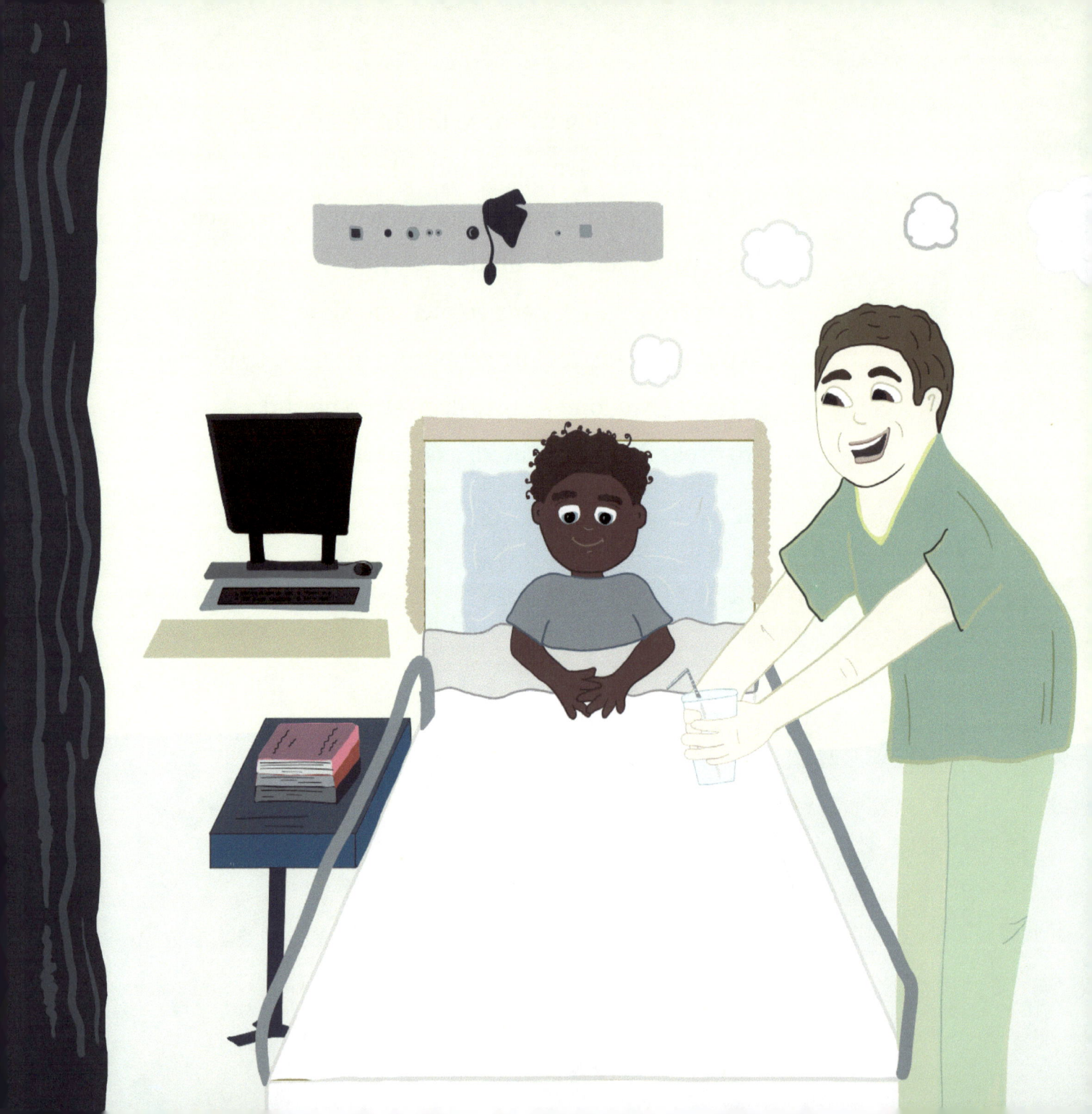

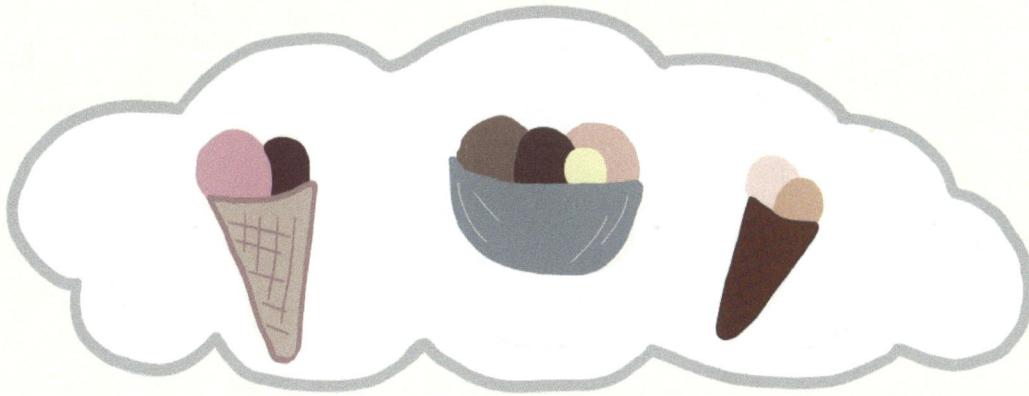

Tommy opened his eyes a bit drowsy and slow,
and a cheery nurse said, "You did great, you know!
Your tonsils are out. It's all done, hooray!
Ice cream is waiting to brighten your day."

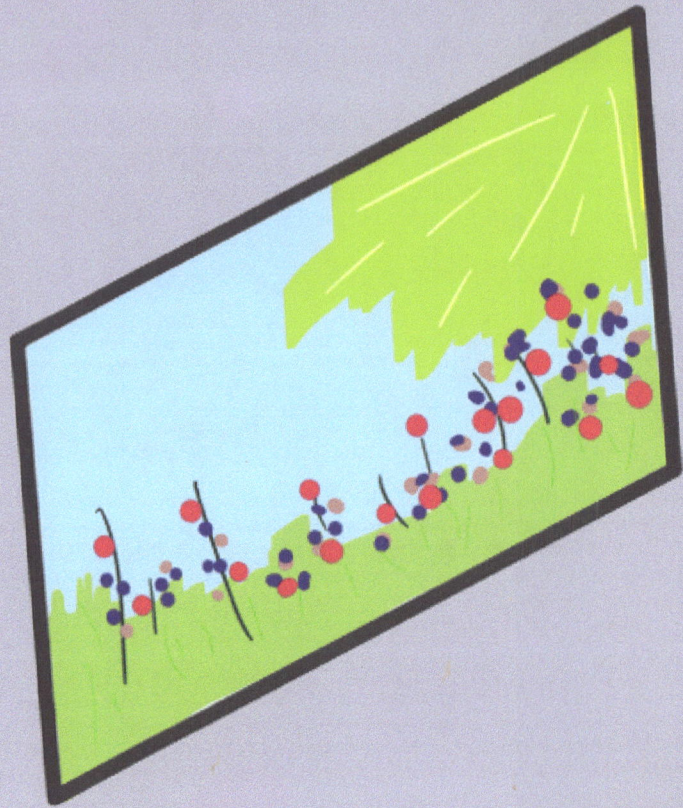

Later in bed, with his teddy bear near,

Tommy grinned wide from ear to ear.

He sipped on cold drinks, feeling cozy and light,

proud that his tonsils had said their goodnight.

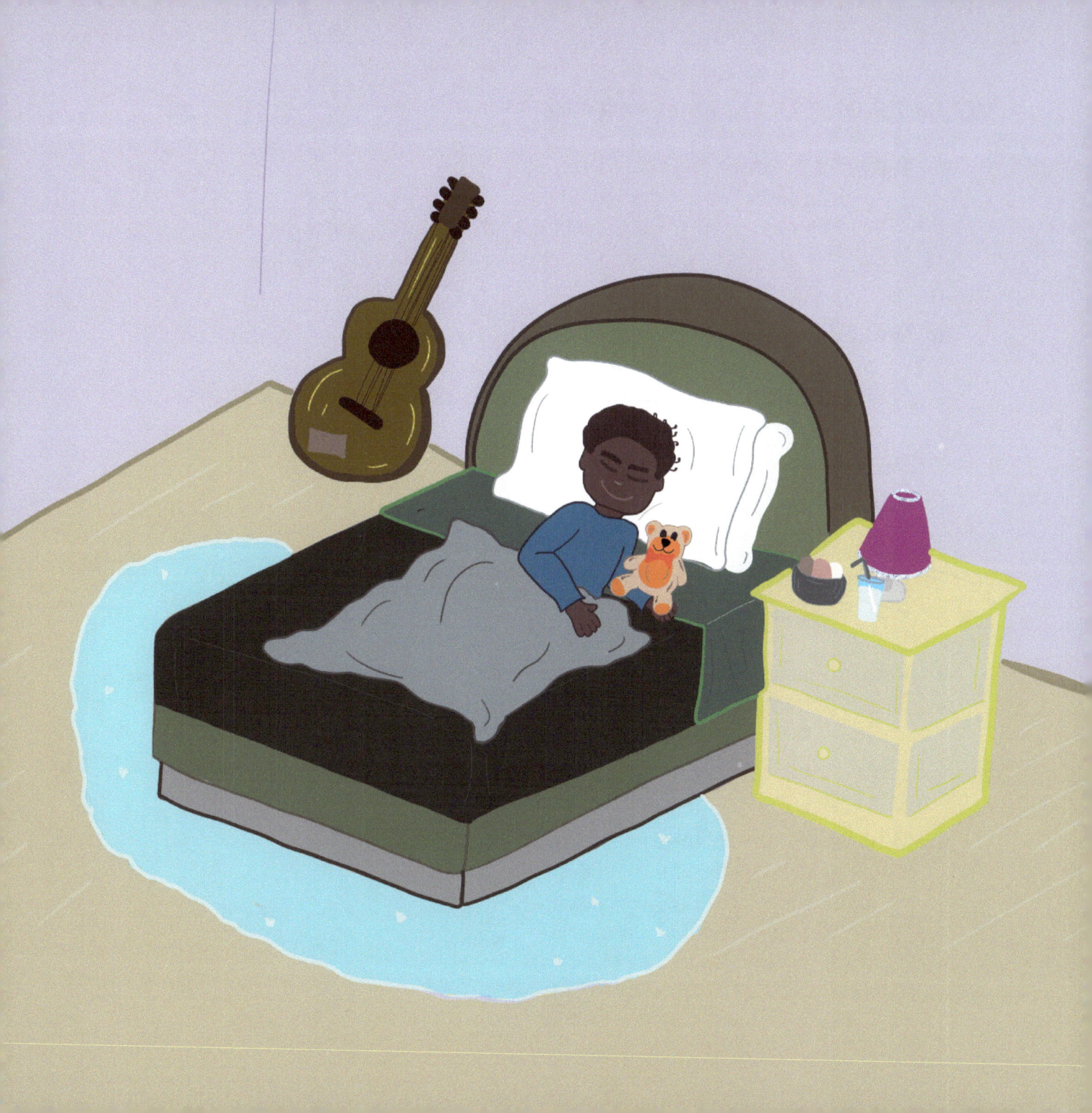

TOMMY'S TONSIL TALES MINI-QUIZ

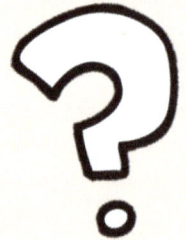

1. **Why did Tommy visit the doctor?**
   a. He had a broken arm that he hurt on the playground
   b. He was snoring when sleeping and kept getting sore throats
   c. He needed a check-up for school with his doctor

2. **What did the doctor suggest to help Tommy with his tonsil trouble?**
   a. Eating lots of candy, especially lollipops
   b. A procedure to have his tonsils taken out (a 'tonsillectomy')
   c. Taking a vacation to go to the beach

3. **What is the role of tonsils in our throat?**
   a. To help us taste our food
   b. To help us sing better
   c. To filter out harmful germs and protect our body

4. **Why do some kids like Tommy need to have their tonsils taken out?**
   a. If they get lots of sore throats or their tonsils get sick often
   b. If they don't like brushing their teeth
   c. If they want to stay up late every night

5. **What did Tommy enjoy doing after his surgery?**
   a. Playing video games all day
   b. Eating sorbet and ice cream
   c. Going on a roller coaster ride

Answers: B, B, C, A, B

Meet the Authors

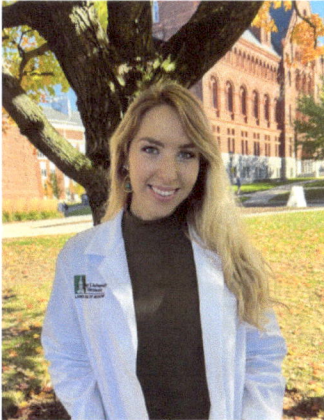

Josephine Yalovitser grew up in Westchester, New York, immersed in Russian culture as the child of immigrants. She discovered her love of the arts early on, with piano and singing at age four. Her work and original compositions have earned national and international recognition, with performances at prestigious venues including Carnegie Hall and Lincoln Center. She went on to study psychology and anthropology at Dartmouth College and will complete her medical degree from the University of Vermont College of Medicine in 2026. Passionate about the intersection of medicine and the arts, Josephine strives to bring creativity, empathy, and a holistic perspective to patient care. Whether through music, medicine, or storytelling, she is committed to healing that honors the full human experience.

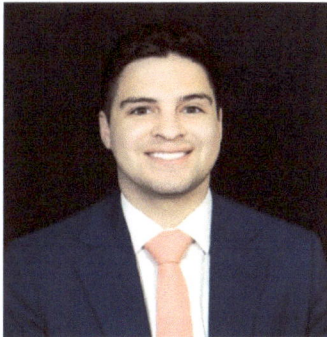

Born in New Haven, Connecticut, in 1997, Christopher Kruglik grew up in the small town of Northford, Connecticut, with his mother and father, two sisters, and two brothers. He went on to receive his Bachelor of Science degree in Biochemistry at the University of Vermont, as well as his Master of Medical Sciences and Master of Public Health. As of 2025, Christopher is currently enrolled in his last year of medical school at the Larner College of Medicine at the University of Vermont. Christopher's clinical interests lie within the sector of the public health realm, pediatrics, and surgery. He is excited to be able to share the *Little Med Minds* book series with his co-author and illustrator to help make children more comfortable and prepared when seeing their physician or getting ready for a surgical procedure.

www.ingramcontent.com/pod-product-compliance
Lightning Source LLC
Chambersburg PA
CBHW061148030426
42335CB00002B/145